Trilsim

Copyright © 2025 by Gerry O Reilly

All rights reserved.

No part of this book may be reproduced or used in any manner without written permission from the copyright owner, except as permitted by law.

Table of Contents

Chapter 1: Introduction

Chapter 2: The Journey

Chapter 3: Reflections

About the Author

The author is a chef, philosopher, and aspiring clinical psychologist with a passion for ethics, history, and science. He writes to inspire critical thinking and meaningful change.

TRILISM

Living an Ethical Life with Mind, Body, and Soul.

A philosophy of Holistic Living, Personal Growth, and Ethical Pragmatism—centred on Mind, Body, and Soul."

Foreword

Trilism: The Way I Live

I didn't set out to write a philosophy. I never dreamed of schools of thought, followers, or legacies. I was trying to live--fully, honestly, and without breaking under the weight of things I never chose. Trilism came from that struggle. From fighting the daily torment that is Crohn's, year after year, decade after decade. From enduring the war within the body, while trying to preserve the mind and soul. From loving others while wrestling with despair. I'm working hard, clinging to integrity, and refusing to let pain turn me bitter or power-hungry.

I never wanted to rule, preach, or profit. I've stepped away from leadership entirely. I am no one's saviour. I walked this road so Trilism would never serve ego -- mine or anyone else's. What's left is a code that cannot be owned. It belongs to you now, if you wish it, and I invite you, the reader, to explore my philosophy.

"Trilism is a philosophy for living well when life is at its worst."

Let me be clear:

- "It is not a religion, but it might offer the solace of one."
- This is not a doctrine, but it might guide like one.
- This is not a revolution, but it might change the world anyway.

Quick question — why did I create Trilism? Because it changed me into the person I needed to become.

So, do you need to change? If your answer is yes, then the next question is — why?

Founder of Trilism

Introduction to Trilism

A Practical Guide for Inner Balance, Resilience, and Meaningful Living —or, to put it plainly: The Way I Live. Forged in Fire and Pain, Bound by Virtue Trilism is not a philosophy born of ease—it was forged in fire. It rose from pain, injustice, isolation, and loss. Its six virtues—Health, Integrity, Resilience, Empathy, Social Harmony, and Authenticity—were not imagined in comfort, but earned through suffering, carved in the dark, and polished by discipline.

- It is peaceful, but not passive.

- Incorruptible, because it has already faced what would shatter others, and chose the harder path of truth.
- It rejects control, hierarchy, and ego. It cannot be bought, branded, or ruled.
- It walks barefoot through fire and still plants seeds of peace.
- This is not a <u>movement</u>.
- This is a rebirth.

Trilism wasn't born from fame, but from friction. It came from the margins of modern life, where survival meets spirit. These six virtues helped me live with dignity when everything else was breaking down. They are not abstract ideals. They are tools—sharpened by reality, tested by hardship, and carried like both blade and balm through the battles of everyday life. Trilism doesn't ask you to be perfect. It invites you to be whole.

- It doesn't demand belief. It asks for reflection.
- It doesn't promise heaven. It helps you build a meaningful now.
- This book isn't about me. (I won't bore you with my life.)
- It's a blueprint for anyone seeking clarity in a chaotic world.

- A guide for the bruised who still reach for beauty.
- If you've found yourself here, welcome. You are not alone.
- And you are not without a path.

Who It's For -

In today's fast-moving and uncertain world, people from all walks of life are searching for a steady, thoughtful way to live. Trilism offers a peaceful, flexible approach to growth—by nurturing the mind, body, and soul in balance.

Trilism is not a religion. It asks nothing of your beliefs, traditions, or culture. Instead, it offers a neutral framework—one that can support anyone on their personal path.

- For students and young people. Trilism brings calm and clarity in a noisy, stressful world. It helps develop confidence, purpose, and resilience in times of learning and change.

- For working adults. Trilism supports focus, self-respect, and emotional balance. It helps maintain integrity in a world that often rewards compromise.
- For parents, caregivers, and older adults. Trilism provides a base for patience, wisdom, and gentle guidance. It encourages peace during responsibility.
- For those in hardship. Trilism is quiet support. No preaching. No pressure. Just calm structure, quiet strength, and

useful direction—without asking you to believe anything you're not ready to.

Whether you study it alone or reflect on it with others, Trilism offers a way to live with strength, honesty, and peace. It doesn't ask for followers—only for people willing to walk with care, compassion, and intent.

A Personal Reckoning

Writing this book has been both a calling and a challenge. I believe in clarity of thought and the effort to live well—but I've wrestled deeply with some ideas along the way.

Take Amor Fati, for instance—the Stoic concept of loving one's fate. How do you explain that to a child who's been abused? Or to a mother working two jobs after losing her partner? Or to someone like me, sick since twenty-one?

I reject the idea that we should embrace suffering blindly. To me, that weakens the spirit. Illness does not hate you. Pain does not conspire. They do not know your name. So why return hatred to something that cannot hear you?

I didn't write this to glorify pain. No one should be expected to embrace hardship without resistance. We must strive to transform, not just endure. You must be patient, yes patient with illness or pain. You need to realize illness, pain or suffering doesn't hate or think of you as an enemy. So, why waste time and energy on something that doesn't even know you exist? Unless someone is causing the pain, illness or suffering but that's completely different. Always remember nothing lasts forever as one of the mottos says.

And maybe, over time, I'll see Amor Fati differently. But Trilism walks a different path—not surrender to fate, but stewardship of self. I couldn't find a philosophy that truly spoke to my experience. So, I built my own. Not to teach, but to survive. And now, to share.

I do not claim that Trilism belongs beside the great philosophical systems of Greece or the East. But I do believe that—if nurtured with reflection and humility—it may help someone survive their darkness with dignity. Because that's what it did for me.

So—Let's begin, shall we?

The Six Core Virtues of Trilism are-

1. Health

2. Integrity

3. Resilience

4. Empathy

5. Social Harmony

6. Authenticity

1. Health First

- Definition: Take care of your body, mind, and soul first—this is the base of a meaningful life.
- Application: Build healthy daily habits like eating well, exercising, sleeping enough, and practicing mindfulness. While some believe the mind is most important, Trilism teaches that a strong body supports a clear mind and a peaceful soul. All three must work together to help a person truly thrive.

Motto: "Health first."

- Example: Leaders who take care of their health often have more energy, focus, and emotional strength. This helps them make wise choices and support others better.

Notes

2. Moral Integrity

- Definition: Do what is right out of a sense of duty, and follow moral rules that support justice, fairness, and respect for everyone.
- Application: Be honest, fair, and open, even when it's hard. Avoid lying or manipulating others, because these actions damage trust and harm communities.

Motto: "There must be balance in life, otherwise chaos ensues."

- Example: Ethical leaders admit their mistakes and tell the truth. By doing so, they build trust and create a respectful environment.

Notes

3. **Emotional Resilience**

- Definition: Stay strong and calm during hard times, while choosing to act with virtue and purpose in response to challenges.

- Application: Build your inner strength and connect with supportive people to get through tough situations. Resilience is not just about surviving—it's about learning and growing from what life throws at you.

Motto: "Get up and get on with it."

- Example: People who keep going after failure often inspire others. Community movements that grow out of struggle show how resilience can lead to real and lasting change.

Notes

4. **Empathetic Decision-Making**

- Definition: Think about how your actions affect others and aim to bring the best to the most people—with kindness, fairness, and care.
- Application: Listen to those who are often ignored and make choices based on empathy and understanding. Let compassion guide how you lead and live.

Motto: "Nothing lasts forever."

- Example: Businesses and groups that care about their workers and communities show this value in action. Decisions made with empathy create fairness and social justice.

Notes

5. Social Harmony

- Definition: Build relationships based on mutual respect, trust, and an understanding that we are all connected.
- Application: Encourage teamwork and open conversation, but don't give up your sense of justice or self-worth. Unlike Amor Fati, which asks people to simply accept what happens, Trilism teaches us to act and push for change when things are unfair.

Motto: "Acceptance is for the weak; we all deserve a better life."

- Example: People who help solve conflicts by lifting up unheard voices and standing against injustice—while still aiming for peace—show the kind of social harmony that Trilism supports one based on justice and active effort, not silent suffering

Notes

6. **Authenticity**

- Definition: Live honestly and stay true to who you really are, with the freedom and courage to take responsibility for your life—even when it means standing alone.

- Application: Show your true values in daily life but also think about how your actions affect others. Being authentic isn't about being selfish—it's about having the strength to live truthfully, even when it's difficult.

Motto: "Be your true self."

- Example: Someone who stays true to themselves during hard times—saying "can't quit, won't quit"—shows real authenticity. Leaders like this often challenge unfair systems and inspire others by simply being real.

Notes

Philosophical Conclusion and Reflection:

My life has been filled with several serious challenges, but through it all, I've tried to find balance—between the mind, body, and soul. Trilism is my way of sharing that balance with others. With this philosophy, I want to encourage people to grow, improve themselves, and live with purpose. Life is hard, but with the right values, we can work toward a life that feels more meaningful and peaceful.

Final Reflection

Trilism gives a clear and practical way to live with purpose and make ethical choices. It's a philosophy that aims for harmony without giving up, honesty without being selfish, and strength without standing still. It might not fit with every old tradition, but I hope it helps people who are trying to understand life's struggles and come out stronger, wiser, and kinder.

Here's your Code of Ethics (COE) for Daily Integration

The values in the COE should be used in everyday life through small, thoughtful actions. Each virtue helps guide personal growth, good choices, and self-reflection. Living by these principles a little each day builds long-term strength and purpose.

Pros and Cons of the COE

Pros:

- Whole-Person Wellness: The COE brings together care for the body, mind, and emotions, helping people become more balanced and complete.

- Ethical Support: It encourages fairness, inclusion, and responsibility, giving people a strong base for making good decisions.
- Useful in Daily Life: The COE gives clear and helpful advice that can be used in real life, supporting steady personal improvement.

Cons:

- Too Strict at Times: The COE might not fit with some personal or cultural beliefs. It may need to be adjusted to avoid feeling too controlling or rigid.
- Emotional Strain: Focusing too much on being strong can make it harder for people to feel safe showing their emotions or asking for help.

- Being True vs. Fitting In: Trying to live honestly and be yourself might not always match with society's rules, which can be tough in more restrictive environments.

Scholarly Framework

The Code of Ethics (COE) can be used in schools, workplaces, and personal life to encourage learning, growth, and strong moral leadership.

Putting COE into Practice in Communities and Leadership

- Wellness Programs: Start activities that help with mindfulness, stress control, and full-body health. These support mental, emotional, and physical well-being.
- Ethics Training: Create a work or group culture based on honesty, responsibility, and clear communication, so ethical behaviour becomes part of daily practice.

- Mentorship: Build support networks where experienced people guide others—emotionally and professionally—sharing wisdom and building strong values.
- Diversity Policies: Make sure everyone has a fair chance, especially those from underrepresented backgrounds. Support equality at every level.
- Community Action: Work with local groups and social causes to push for real change and speak up for those who are often unheard.

Final Thoughts: A Call for Ethical Pragmatism

The Code of Ethics isn't a fixed set of rules or a religious system—it's a living, flexible guide. It offers a way to find balance, fairness, and personal growth. This philosophy is built on the idea that the world doesn't need more empty ideas. It needs honest, strong, and caring people who live with empathy and truth.

My philosophy is for those who believe that simply accepting suffering isn't always right—especially when we have the power to make things better. What the world truly needs is action. With the COE, we can take that action.

"Acceptance is for who?" Answer: Not for you.

The COE can be used in schools, workplaces, and personal reflection. It fosters ethical discussion, supports mental wellness, and encourages inclusive problem-solving across generations.

Daily Plan for Integration:

1. Health First

- Definition: Make physical, mental, and emotional well-being a priority because they are the foundation of a happy and successful life.
- Application: Develop daily habits that support your health, such as good nutrition, exercise, rest, and mindfulness. A healthy body, mind, and spirit are necessary to live with integrity and take action. Contrary to what some philosophers believe, the body must be well cared for so the mind can work at its best.

Motto: "Health first."

- Real-World Example: Leaders who focus on their own health set a good example for their teams and communities. This leads to healthier, more productive societies. Encouraging work-life balance and mental health programs helps create an environment where everyone can succeed.

2. Moral Integrity

- Definition: Act with a strong sense of responsibility, following universal moral rules that promote justice and fairness.
- Application: Treat everyone with respect and fairness. Always think about how your actions affect others. Listen to marginalized voices and support policies that encourage equality.

Motto: "There must be balance in life; otherwise, chaos ensues."

- Ethical change. Ethical decision-making begins with the courage to admit mistakes and correct them without dishonesty.

3. Emotional Resilience

- Definition: Build inner strength and calm when facing difficulties, understanding the importance of both personal and group growth.
- Application: Focus on personal development and doing the right thing, while also accepting help from others and acknowledging things that are beyond your

control. Resilience means growing stronger through challenges, not staying stuck.

Motto: "Get up and get on with it."

- Real-World Example: Activists who experience personal loss but continue working for social change show the strength of resilience. Their ability to keep going despite hardships inspires others to join the fight for justice.

4. Empathetic Decision-Making

- Definition: Think about the effects of your actions, aiming to do the best while respecting diversity.
- Application: Serve others by making choices that focus on the well-being of the

whole group. Include the experiences of marginalized communities in decision-making to create fair and equal outcomes.

Motto: "Nothing lasts forever.

- Real-World Example: Organizations that care for their employees and communities demonstrate empathetic decision-making. This might include policies that offer healthcare, equal opportunities, and fair wages.

5. Social Harmony

- Definition: Build relationships based on trust and respect, understanding that we all share a common humanity and that diverse viewpoints are valuable.

- Application: Work together through discussions, solve conflicts with understanding, and respect different perspectives. Aim to improve both your own life and your community's situation. While we can't always change the world, we have the power to make our lives and society better through thoughtful actions.

Motto: "Acceptance is for the weak; everyone has the right to a better life."

- Real-World Example: Community leaders who focus on amplifying marginalized voices and challenge social injustice with empathy and accountability show how social harmony can create positive change.

6. Authenticity

- Definition: Live in a way that is true to yourself, accepting your freedom, responsibility, and accountability.
- Application: Be true to your values and beliefs, even when others might disagree. Authenticity is not about being selfish; it is about having the courage to stand by your principles.

Motto: "Be your true self."

- Real-World Example: People who face challenges authentically—whether as activists, artists, or leaders—challenge societal norms and fight for justice, inspiring others to act with honesty and integrity.

Conclusion

The Code of Ethics (COE) is not a strict, authoritarian, or religious rulebook, but rather a flexible and evolving guide. It encourages people to live balanced lives, contribute to their communities, and act with integrity. At its core, Trilism aims to inspire people to practice ethical pragmatism—making decisions based on the values of health, integrity, resilience, empathy, harmony, and authenticity. Trilism offers a moral compass that helps individuals navigate their lives with strength, clarity, and purpose, while avoiding the limitations of rigid ideologies.

Let this philosophy guide you, and always remember: "Acceptance is for who? Not for you."

★★★★★★★★★★★★

Daily Integration Plan for Individuals.

1. MORNING RITUAL (Upon Waking – 6.00am to 9:00 AM)

Virtues: Health · Integrity · Resilience

- Wake with Purpose
- Open the day with this spoken or silent intention:
- "Today I will live with clarity, courage, and care."

Hydrate and Nourish

- A high-protein, balanced breakfast supports both mind and body. Respect your health as a sacred duty. Make as much homemade food as possible. No news, no technology, just peace and stillness.

Body Activation (10–15 min)

- Gentle movement—stretching, walking, or bodyweight exercises. Connect to your vessel.

Integrity Journal (5 min)

- Write your answers:
- What will I do today that aligns with my deeper values?
- Where do I risk betraying myself, and how will I resist?

Before you leave the home please do this as I do as often as I can:

- Just take one minute at your front door and breathe. Think to yourself - "I will meet nice people and some horrible people. But I will be the good person I actually wish to meet today ".

2. MIDDAY PRACTICE (12:00 PM – 2:00 PM)

Virtues: Authenticity · Social Harmony
- Authentic Check-In (1 min)
- Stop. Breathe. Ask:

- Am I being sincere in my words, actions, and presence?
- Am I living my truth or performing a role?

- Conscious Communication (1 interaction minimum)
- Speak to someone with intention: listen fully, respond with care. One moment of pure presence can ripple.

Midday Nourishment

- Eat with awareness—no distractions.
- See food not as consumption, but as communion with the world.
- When you sleep, you sleep. When you walk, you walk.
- So, when you eat—you eat.
- Honour this moment as sacred. Take it just for you—no technology, no noise, only stillness and sustenance.

3. AFTERNOON FLOW (3:00 PM – 6:00 PM)

Virtues: Resilience · Health · Integrity

- Focused Work or Craft (1–2 hours)
- Dedicate time to something you believe in—creative, physical, intellectual. This builds both resilience and dignity.

Resilience Checkpoint

- Ask: What challenged me today? How did I respond? How can I grow from it?

Body Reset (15 min)

- Movement, fresh air, sunlight—restore your physical energy.

4. EVENING REFLECTION (7:00 PM – 10:00 PM)

Virtues: Empathy · Authenticity · Social Harmony

Empathy Offering

- Reach out to one person with kindness—check in, send a voice note, offer help. A small act strengthens social harmony.

Reflective Writing (10 min)

- Where did I act in virtue today?
- Where did I fall short, and how can I do better tomorrow?

- What emotion did I avoid—and what truth lay beneath it?

Gratitude + Letting Go

- Whisper or write three gratitude's, and one thing to release.

5. NIGHT RITUAL (Before Sleep)

Virtue: Health

Digital Silence (60 min before bed)

- Honour your mind's need for peace. Unplug and allow stillness.

Rest as a Sacred Act

- Say: "I've done what I could. The rest will wait. I return to the Source."

(The Source in Trilism is what restores you—call it the deeper Self, the flow of life, nature, the cosmos, or simply the great stillness that holds all things. You define it. What matters is the return)

Optional Weekly Additions:

Weekly Solitude (1 hour minimum)
No input. No output. Just you, nature, and stillness.

Connection Circle (Weekly)

Share your journey—virtues, struggles, and growth—with a fellow Trilism practitioner or trusted companion.

Monthly Reflection

Rate how you embodied each virtue (1–10).

Set intentions to restore balance where needed.

Leaders in Governance According to COE

Definition

Governance, within the framework of Code of Ethics (COE), is not merely the exercise of leadership and policymaking; it is the ethical orchestration of communal well-being, justice, and sustainable development. Guided by the six core virtues—Health, Integrity, Resilience, Empathy, Social Harmony, and Authenticity—COE governance emphasizes both ethical stewardship and practical action to ensure a society that thrives holistically.

Core Principles of COE Governance

1. Health as a Public Priority

Governance must prioritize the holistic health—physical, mental, and environmental—of its population as the cornerstone of a sustainable and thriving society.

2. Virtue-Driven Leadership

All leaders and institutions must exemplify the six core virtues in both their personal and public lives. Ethics must always precede efficiency.

3. Resilience in Policy and Crisis Management

Institutions must be structured to adapt and evolve through crises, ensuring the safeguarding of rights and communal trust in the face of disruption.

4. Participatory Decision-Making

Governance is a shared social process. Citizens must be empowered to influence laws, policies, and norms that affect their lives, ensuring democratic and inclusive representation.

5. Compassionate Administration

Empathy should inform the tone and intent of laws. Policies must be measured not only by their legality but also by their humanity and capacity to serve the common good.

6. Transparent and Accountable Systems

Integrity and Authenticity demand open records, public access to information, and clear accountability mechanisms at all levels of authority.

7. Social Harmony and Inclusivity

Governance must serve as a bridge, not a wall. It should actively mend divisions, encourage diversity, and foster inclusive civic spaces.

Governance Mottos Derived from COE

"Lead not for dominion, but for devotion."
"The strength of a law lies in its justice, not its enforcement."

"Authority must mirror the ethics of those it serves."

The Soul of Governance

In the COE view, governance is not a mechanism of control but a living reflection of a society's moral spine. Leadership is not claimed—it is entrusted. Power is not an entitlement—it is a responsibility grounded in virtue and answerable to the whole.

Governance in Practice

1. Ethical Councils

Advisory bodies comprising ethicists, community leaders, and citizen delegates ensure that new laws and policies align with COE principles.

2. Public Health Mandates

Regular audits of public health initiatives ensure that they remain aligned with the Health virtue, emphasizing proactive care and well-being.

3. Empathy Reviews

Periodic citizen-feedback cycles assess the emotional and social impact of major policies, ensuring they contribute to the collective well-being.

4. Social Harmony Indexes

Governments assess societal well-being not just through GDP, but by using indices that measure inclusion, trust, and conflict resolution.

Global Relevance

COE governance is adaptable across political systems. It does not seek to replace democracy, socialism, or any existing system, but to elevate any structure through ethical refinement. It is pragmatic idealism—balancing visionary values with real-world applications to foster global justice and harmony. Application of COE Governance in Leadership and Society

1. Health First

- Definition: Prioritize physical, mental, and emotional well-being as the foundation of a fulfilled and successful life.
- Application: Encourage health-centred habits, including proper nutrition, exercise, rest, and mindfulness, to foster resilience and clarity in decision-making. A healthy population is better equipped to thrive in society and make ethical decisions.

Motto: "Health first."

- Example: Leaders who maintain their own health inspire others to do the same, resulting in a more resilient and productive society.

2. Moral Integrity

- Definition: Act with a strong sense of duty, adhering to universal moral principles that uphold justice and equity.
- Application: Leaders and citizens must uphold fairness and respect in all interactions, addressing systemic inequalities through inclusive policies and ensuring transparency.

Motto: "There must be balance in life, otherwise chaos ensues."

- Example: Leaders who prioritize transparency and accountability foster trust and actively address systemic inequalities.

3. Emotional Resilience

- Definition: Cultivate inner strength and composure in the face of adversity, recognizing the importance of growth, both personal and collective.
- Application: Respond to challenges with composure, relying on community support and proactive strategies to overcome hardships.

Motto: "Get up and get on with it."

- Example: Individuals who maintain resilience in adversity inspire others to persist, especially in social justice movements.

4. Empathetic Decision-Making

- Definition: Evaluate actions based on their consequences, striving for the greatest good for all while embracing diversity.
- Application: Serve the collective needs of society by prioritizing empathy and collaboration, ensuring fair outcomes for marginalized communities. No one is left behind.

Motto: "Nothing lasts forever."

- Example: Organizations that prioritize the well-being of their employees and communities, addressing inequalities through fair policies, demonstrate empathetic leadership.

5. Social Harmony

- Definition: Build relationships based on mutual trust and respect, recognizing our shared humanity and the value of diverse perspectives.
- Application: Resolve conflicts through understanding and cooperation, fostering dialogues that respect and embrace diverse identities.

Motto: "Acceptance is for the weak; we all have the right to a better life."

- Example: Communities that prioritize inclusivity and conflict resolution create harmonious environments that celebrate diversity.

6. Authenticity

- Definition: Embrace individual freedom and authenticity by aligning choices with personal values, while recognizing their impact on others.
- Application: Leaders must take responsibility for their actions and the consequences of those choices. An inclusive environment should be cultivated, allowing diverse identities to thrive while

balancing personal expression with communal responsibility.

Motto: "Be your true self."

- Example: Leaders who embody authenticity inspire others to pursue their true selves and advocate for social justice and equity, creating spaces where everyone can express their identity without fear of judgment.

Final Thoughts

The Code of Ethics (GCOE) is a living framework, not a rigid authoritarian doctrine. It encourages personal responsibility, ethical leadership, and societal well-being. By focusing on small, intentional actions and fostering a mindful approach to decisions, individuals and communities can integrate COE's principles into their daily lives. As we work toward a more ethical and harmonious society, we must remember that health and well-being are the bedrock of all virtues. A just society starts with ethical people who prioritize health, integrity, resilience, empathy, social harmony and authenticity. **"No one is unseen."**

The Daily Praxis of Ethical Leadership
Applied Governance Through COE Virtues

True leadership is not episodic—it is rhythmic. It arises not only in great decisions, but in ordinary moments governed by extraordinary awareness. The following daily framework serves as a compass for leaders who seek to embody COE principles not just in policy, but in presence. These practices cultivate internal integrity, ethical clarity, and communal trust. To govern well is first to govern oneself.

1. DAWN DISCIPLINE (5:30–8:00 AM)

Virtues: Integrity · Health · Resilience

- Silent Intention (2 minutes)
- "I serve not for power, but for peace. I rule not by command, but by example."

Physical Awakening

- Exercise, breathwork, or martial movement. A strong leader governs from a strong vessel.

Integrity Forecast (Journal Prompt)

- What decisions today will test my ethics?
- What hidden agendas must I resist?

- How do I remain principled without becoming rigid?

Ethical Briefing (15 min)
- Review policies, memos, or strategy only through the lens of virtue. Ask: Does this respect the soul of the people?

2. MORNING ACTION (9:00–12:00)

Virtues: Authenticity · Integrity · Social Harmony
- Transparent Leadership Touchpoint
- Hold one meeting or communication that exemplifies openness. Speak plainly, without pretence.
- Lead as if every word were public.

Integrity Filter

- Before each major action:
- Is this fair?
- Is this necessary?
- Would I still choose it if I were the lowest person affected by it?

Team Listening Session (15–30 min)

- One period each week dedicated to hearing concerns—without defending or deflecting. Just listen.

3. MIDDAY ALIGNMENT (12:30–2:00 PM)

Virtues: Health · Empathy

- Silent Meal (15–20 min)
- Eat alone or in silence. Reflect on stewardship:
- Am I nourishing myself like someone who must care for others?

Empathy Calibration

- Read or review one real story—an email, a case, a plea. Sit with it. Feel what it would be like to live under your decisions.

4. AFTERNOON RESOLVE (2:00–5:00 PM)

Virtues: Resilience · Integrity

- Hard Decisions with Soft Hands
- Govern with discipline, not cruelty. When rejecting, do so with dignity. When punishing, do so with humility.

Resilience Note

- Log one moment where you could have collapsed into cynicism—but didn't. That is victory.

Leadership Accountability Session (Weekly)

- Invite feedback from your team. No defensiveness.

- The leader who cannot be questioned is no longer leading.

5. EVENING RECKONING (6:00–9:00 PM)

Virtues: Authenticity · Empathy · Social Harmony

Daily Reckoning Log

- Where did I uphold virtue under pressure?
- Where did I slip—and why?
- Whose voice did I neglect?
- Was my leadership a mirror of my soul or a mask?
- Offer a Restorative Act
- End your public day by performing or planning one act to restore trust, right a wrong, or uplift a soul.

6. NIGHT RETURN (Before Sleep)

Virtue: Health

Stillness Ritual

- No media. No decisions. Just stillness and breath. Return to yourself.
- "Governance is not mine—it is the duty I carry for others."

Optional Weekly Components

Virtue Audit (Weekly – 1 hr)

Review all six virtues in relation to your leadership. Score 1–10. Ask: Am I slipping into performance or deepening into presence?

Public Transparency Statement (Monthly)

Share one area where you grew, failed, or changed your stance. Normalize ethical evolution.

Shadow Review (Quarterly)

Bring in someone you trust to challenge your blind spots. No echo chambers.

Closing Reflection

Ethical governance is not a mask worn in the public square; it is the interior discipline of living by principle when no one is watching. As the sun sets on each day, let the leader not ask, "Was I obeyed?" but rather, "Was I just? Was I true?" In the silence of night, let peace be the reward of conscience, and may every return to stillness renew the vow: I lead not to rule, but to serve.

Remember: "The plan doesn't make it great; what we have and work for together is what makes the plan great."

Trilism: A Peaceful and Incorruptible Ethos Summary of Structure and Virtue Integrity

Trilism is a virtue-centred philosophy that harmonizes the Mind, Body, and Soul, anchored in six cardinal virtues: Health, Integrity, Resilience, Empathy, Social Harmony, and Authenticity. It offers no hierarchy, no doctrine, no master—only a living code of conscious conduct for individuals, communities, and ethical leaders.

Its peaceful nature emerges from decentralization. No leaders. No coercion. No dogma. Every adherent governs themselves by conscience and virtue, not by force or reward.

Its incorruptibility is guarded through voluntary transparency, rigorous self-reflection, and the deliberate refusal to pursue power for its own sake.

- Trilism is **not** a movement.
- It is a way of being.
- It cannot be owned, sold, or controlled—only practiced.

Peacefulness

Trilism fosters peace through its six virtues, especially by emphasizing health, empathy, and harmony. These cultivate a world where individuals tend their well-being, respect one another, and prioritize cooperation over competition.

Yet, peace is not passivity. A potential shadow of harmony is the suppression of dissent or avoidance of necessary conflict. Trilism must therefore embed constructive conflict resolution and open dialogue into its culture to ensure peace remains vibrant, not stagnant.

Incorruptibility

Trilism's structural immunity to corruption lies in its reliance on Moral Integrity, Authenticity, and Resilience. These virtues ensure that decisions are guided by truth, not ego, and that accountability is internal, not imposed.

However, rigid morality without flexibility can lead to ethical paralysis in complex contexts. Trilism must remain grounded in ethical pragmatism—adapting without compromising core principles.

Virtue Analysis: Strengths & Tensions

1. Health First

Pros: Cultivates vitality, clarity, and long-term resilience; reduces societal strain.

Cons: Risk of health perfectionism; may overshadow other forms of fulfilment (e.g., art, rest).

2. Moral Integrity

Pros: Builds trust and addresses injustice through principled living.

Cons: Rigid application may lack nuance and strain pluralistic communities.

3. Emotional Resilience

Pros: Equips individuals to thrive under pressure and recover from hardship.

Cons: May overemphasize strength, undervaluing vulnerability and the legitimacy of emotional pain.

4. Empathetic Decision-Making

Pros: Ensures fairness, equity, and connection across diverse groups.

Cons: Can delay critical decisions and cause emotional fatigue in complex leadership contexts.

5. Social Harmony

Pros: Reduces conflict and builds inclusive, safe communities.

Cons: Risk of avoiding necessary confrontations or stifling honest dissent.

6. Authenticity

Pros: Invites honest expression and meaningful contribution to society.

Cons: Radical authenticity may clash with social norms, causing friction or alienation.

Trilism vs. Dualism

Trilism offers a deeper and more balanced view of human nature than Plato's classical Dualism. While Dualism divides human beings into two separate parts—the mind (reason) and the body (flesh)—Trilism sees us as made up of three interconnected elements: mind, body, and soul. In Trilism, the mind represents thought, learning, and awareness. The body represents health, action, and physical presence. The soul is the moral and emotional core—the part that feels, cares, and connects us to meaning and purpose. These three elements are not in conflict; they are meant to support and strengthen each other.

Why Trilism Offers More

Whole-Person Wisdom: By uniting mind, body, and soul, Trilism gives a fuller understanding of what it means to live well. It encourages people to think clearly, live healthily, and act with kindness and conscience.

Balanced Growth: Trilism doesn't just focus on one part of life. It supports mental clarity, physical well-being, and spiritual depth—helping individuals grow while also caring for the community

Inner Harmony, Outer Peace: A person who nourishes all three elements is more likely to make ethical choices, remain resilient under stress, and live with integrity. Trilism creates space for both personal fulfilment and social harmony.

Challenges of Trilism

Abstract Ideas: Not everyone finds it easy to understand or work with ideas like "soul." Unlike the body, which is visible, and the mind, which is logical, the soul is often felt rather than defined—this makes it hard to measure or teach clearly.

Subjective Experience: Every person experiences their inner world differently. What one person calls "spiritual," another may see as emotional or intuitive. This means Trilism must stay open, flexible, and non-dogmatic to remain practical and inclusive.

Conclusion

Trilism stands as a fundamentally peaceful and corruption-resistant philosophy. Rooted in six guiding virtues—Health, Integrity, Resilience, Empathy, Social Harmony, and Authenticity—it provides a moral and practical foundation for fostering ethical leadership, personal growth, and communal well-being

Its strength lies in its commitment to virtue-driven self-governance and decentralized responsibility, ensuring that no individual holds unchecked power and that every follower is accountable to conscience rather than command. This structure cultivates trust, compassion, and mutual respect, vital qualities for any just and stable society.

However, for Trilism to remain effective in complex, real-world scenarios, it must embrace ethical pragmatism—the ability to apply virtue flexibly without compromising it. In situations where ideals meet uncertainty or moral ambiguity, pragmatic reasoning helps preserve the spirit of virtue while adapting to context. Furthermore, incorporating transparent checks and balances, such as virtue audits or peer accountability, would enhance its resilience and guard against ethical drift.

In sum, Trilism offers more than a philosophical ideal—it presents a workable model for ethical living and governance, grounded in holistic well-being and collective responsibility. As a living philosophy, it empowers individuals and communities alike to build a world that is not only functional, but profoundly humane.

Governance Through Trilism: Practical Models

A governance system rooted in Trilism is guided not by dominance or partisanship, but by the ethical integration of Health, Integrity, Resilience, Empathy, Social Harmony, and Authenticity. Rather than imposing rigid ideologies, Trilist governance seeks to nurture a just, compassionate, and sustainable society. Below are key mechanisms that embody these ideals in practical terms:

1. Health-Centric Policies
    - Role: The principle of "Health First" ensures that governance begins with the well-being of the people. This includes not only

physical health but also mental, emotional, and social health.

- Functionality: Trilist governments would proactively invest in preventive care, public health education, and supportive infrastructure that sustains long-term health outcomes. Policies would promote balanced living, including mental health support, access to clean environments, and encouragement of physical vitality.

- Example: A Trilist government might establish nationwide wellness initiatives—such as subsidized access to nutritious food, mental health counselling in schools and workplaces, and community fitness programs—aimed at cultivating long-term societal resilience.

2. Ethical Councils for Oversight

- Role: Their primary duty would be to review proposed policies and decisions through the lens of Trilism's six virtues.
- Functionality: Rather than acting as partisan critics, they would function as moral auditors, ensuring that governance remains empathetic, transparent, and authentically aligned with the public good.
- Example: If a healthcare policy disproportionately impacts marginalized communities, the Ethical Council would assess its virtue alignment, offering revisions that prioritize fairness, dignity, and access—thus harmonizing legislative intent with lived reality.

3. Transparent and Participatory Governance

- Role: In a Trilist system, transparency and active citizen participation are not luxuries but imperatives. Governance must be visible, understandable, and accessible to all, ensuring that power remains accountable and grounded in Integrity.
- Functionality: Through open records, public forums, and digital access to legislative proceedings, citizens are empowered to understand, question, and contribute to the decisions that shape their lives. This model fosters civic trust and reinforces Authenticity in leadership.
- Example: Public "Empathy Reviews"—systematic feedback loops inviting marginalized or underrepresented groups to assess policy outcomes—could become

standard practice. These reviews ensure that laws evolve in alignment with diverse lived experiences, enhancing Social Harmony and ethical inclusivity.

4. Conflict Resolution and Social Harmony
- Role: True Social Harmony is not the absence of conflict, but the presence of systems that facilitate respectful discourse and equitable resolutions. Conflict, when addressed constructively, becomes a source of insight and cohesion.
- Functionality: Trilist governance would support community-based mediation councils and dialogue forums that elevate emotional intelligence and collective problem-solving. These mechanisms

prevent escalation, foster mutual understanding, and prioritize Empathy as a civic tool.

- Example: A neighbourhood mediation body, composed of trusted local members and trained facilitators, could handle disputes ranging from housing concerns to intergroup tensions. By creating safe spaces for honest dialogue, such councils would embody Resilience and Harmony, transforming potential divisions into opportunities for unity.

5. Authenticity in Leadership and Policy
- Role: In a Trilist framework, authenticity is the moral compass of leadership. Leaders

are not merely administrators of policy—they are embodiments of the values they champion. Their words and actions must reflect inner coherence, moral clarity, and public accountability.

- Functionality: Authentic leaders communicate transparently about their goals, challenges, and decision-making processes. Rather than concealing motives or deflecting responsibility, they demonstrate ethical congruence—acting in ways that resonate with both their conscience and the collective virtues of the community.
- Example: In the face of complex issues like environmental sustainability, a Trilist leader would not simply announce a policy

shift. They would articulate the ethical dilemmas, disclose the long-term vision, and invite public reflection. This form of values-based governance deepens trust and cultivates an informed, morally invested citizenry.

Ethical Applications of Trilism: Real-World Integration

Trilism is not just a philosophy—it is a practical ethical compass that can guide individuals and communities through daily life and institutional operations. Grounded in the six core virtues, its applications span personal conduct and organizational culture.

Daily Ethical Decisions Guided by Virtue

1. Health First: Individuals would prioritize physical and mental well-being through intentional routines that balance work, rest, and self-care. For example, integrating regular physical activity, healthy eating, and mindfulness practices cultivates long-term resilience and emotional stability.

- Moral Integrity: Ethical behaviour would be embedded into daily interactions. Whether it's admitting an error at work or standing firm against dishonest practices, actions would reflect fairness, honesty, and responsibility—even when inconvenient.

- Emotional Resilience: Rather than reacting impulsively to stress or setbacks, people would develop tools such as reflection, emotional regulation, and community connection. This approach fosters inner strength without denying vulnerability.

- Empathetic Decision-Making: Individuals would make decisions not only for personal benefit but with consideration of their broader impact—especially on vulnerable groups. This might mean advocating for someone's voice in a group setting or adjusting a plan to better accommodate others' needs.

- Social Harmony: Even in disagreement, Trilist practitioners would engage in civil dialogue, seek mutual understanding, and aim for peaceful solutions. Volunteering, participating in local initiatives, or mediating small disputes all contribute to a more cohesive society.

- Authenticity: Each person would align choices with their deeper values. Whether selecting a profession, engaging in activism, or simply expressing an honest opinion, they would live with integrity and courage—regardless of external pressures.

2. Organizational Ethics Rooted in Trilism

- Organizations—corporate, nonprofit, or governmental—can use Trilism to establish a culture of ethical excellence, resilience, and inclusivity.

- Health-Centred Workplaces: Companies would prioritize employee wellness through flexible schedules, mental health resources, ergonomic spaces, and wellness programs that affirm the value of human dignity and long-term vitality.

- Transparency and Accountability: Institutional trust would be built through consistent communication, clear ethics policies, and stakeholder inclusion. Regular audits, open forums, and values-based leadership training would ensure decisions remain aligned with Trilism's principles.

- Resilience Through Adaptation: In a crisis, Trilist organizations wouldn't resort to reactive measures alone. Instead, they'd foster creativity, foresight, and communal strength—adapting not just to survive, but to grow ethically and sustainably.

- Social Responsibility and the Virtue of Harmony

Trilism encourages companies and institutions to embrace social responsibility by adopting inclusive practices, promoting diversity, and actively contributing to community well-being. This is a direct reflection of the virtues of Social Harmony and Empathy. When organizations consider the impact of their operations on people and society, they help build a more compassionate, cooperative, and equitable world.

Conclusion: Trilism as a Blueprint for Ethical Societies

Trilism offers a well-rounded, peaceful ethical framework that values the unity of mind, body, and soul. It promotes personal balance, collective well-being, and principled leadership. By applying its core virtues—Health, Integrity, Resilience, Empathy, Social Harmony, and Authenticity—to everyday choices and public policies, Trilism serves as a guide for creating ethical and resilient societies.

Through practical tools such as ethical councils, transparent governance, and health-first policies, Trilism can reshape both individual behaviour and institutional structures. It minimizes corruption by placing empathy, authenticity, and accountability at the heart of leadership and decision-making.

In an ever-changing world, Trilism provides a flexible yet principled foundation. It empowers people and communities to live with purpose, act with compassion, and govern with wisdom—offering not just a philosophy, but a viable path toward a more just and sustainable future.

The Trilism Manifesto

By Gerry, Philosopher of Mind, Body, and Soul

We stand at the threshold of a new era—an age that demands clarity, compassion, and courage. In a fragmented world of fleeting ideals, Trilism emerges as a guiding compass, forged from the enduring elements of human existence: Mind, Body, and Soul.

Trilism is not merely a philosophy. It is a code of life—a conscious way of being, grounded in six essential virtues that illuminate the path to personal fulfilment and collective harmony:

Health First, for the body is the vessel through which all-purpose flows.

Moral Integrity, to anchor us in truth, even when compromise tempts.

Emotional Resilience, to endure, adapt, and rise with dignity from life's trials.

Empathetic Decision-Making, to govern with both reason and compassion.

Social Harmony, to nurture unity without silencing individuality.

Authenticity, for truth to self is the genesis of truth to others.

We, the Trilists, believe that well-being is a moral imperative, not a privilege. That authenticity is not rebellion, but alignment with one's deeper truth. That empathy is not weakness, but the purest form of strength. And that to heal society, we must first integrate ourselves.

Trilism stands for a world where ethical pragmatism replaces hollow idealism, where the well-being of the community carries equal weight with individual success, and where each person is invited—not to conform, but to evolve.

This is not a utopian fantasy. This is a practical ethic for real people, living real lives in real time. Trilism is not a dogma—it is a living philosophy.

To live as a Trilist is to pledge oneself to something greater than convenience. It is to walk the path of virtue with humility and fire. It is to see the human being not as a problem to be solved, but as a harmony to be tuned.

Let this be our declaration:

That we are whole, not fragmented.
That we are responsible, not resigned.
That we are free—not in the pursuit of self above all, but in service to meaning, integrity, and soul.
There is no pride, and there is no ego, for pride and ego are contrary to the heart of Trilism.

There is no "me," and there is no "you"—there is only us.

Let this be our offering to the future:

A philosophy not for the few, but for the many.

Not for the powerful, but for the principled.

Not for the moment, but for the ages.

We are the Trilists.

We choose Health, Integrity, Resilience, Empathy, Social Harmony, and Authenticity.

We choose Mind, Body, and Soul—as one.

We choose not to control humanity—but to evolve it.

I am the founder and the first, but not the leader.

I do not dictate. I do not command

Will you become a Trilist—

To build a better world,

A more just society,

And a life of peace, purpose, and truth for all?

Guide for the Next Trilist

1. Learn and Embody Trilism

- Understand the Six Virtues: Dive deep into their meaning. Reflect on how they shape your life and actions.
- Live Mind-Body-Soul Harmony: Trilism is not merely a belief system—it is a lived practice. Align your actions with your essence.
- Read the Manifesto Daily for the first month: Make it your guiding oath. Internalize it, for it is your compass on this journey.

2. Own It Personally

- Write Your Why: Journal your reasons for choosing Trilism. Reflect on its impact on your life—daily.
- Share Your Journey: Let others know how Trilism has transformed your health, mindset, relationships, and choices.
- Create Your Trilist Story: Your personal story is a living testament to the philosophy's power.

3. Be a Voice, Not an Echo

- Speak in Your Own Voice: Share Trilism using your language, your metaphors. Make it your own.

- Don't Just Repeat: Reflect on and evolve Trilism. Each Trilist contributes to the growth of this philosophy by interpreting it with sincerity and authenticity.

  Bring It to Your Work: Whether you are a teacher, healer, artist, or speaker—integrate Trilism naturally into your professional life.

4. Invite Others, Gently

- Share, Don't Preach: Say: "There's a philosophy that changed my life. It's called Trilism. Can I share it with you?"
- Introduce the Manifesto and Six Virtues: Ask: "Which of these resonates most with you?"

- Let Curiosity Lead: Encourage exploration without pressure. Let others come to it with an open heart.

5. Create Visible Acts of Trilism
   - Be Known for Your Actions: Let kindness, clarity, health, and truth shine through in everything you do.
   - Practice Compassion: Help others, mediate conflicts, live authentically, and embody integrity.
   - Say It Out Loud: Boldly state, "This is what being a Trilist means to me." Your example will inspire others.

6. Build a Small Circle

- Start with a Seed Group: Invite one or two like-minded individuals to begin your first "Trilist Seed Group.
- Meet Regularly: Discuss how you apply the virtues in your daily lives—weekly or monthly gatherings are ideal.
- Make It Sacred: Keep it informal, but rooted in practice, not perfection.

7. Protect the Spirit

- Guard the Integrity of Trilism: Trilism is not a trend or product—it is a sacred path.
- Stay True to the Essence: Never let it be hijacked by ego, politics, or profit.

- Honour the Founder's Spirit: "I am not a leader. I do not dictate." This keeps Trilism pure, noble, and accessible to all.

A Call to the Next Trilist

By stepping into the role of the next Trilist, you are not just following a philosophy—you are becoming the first branch of the tree. You show the world that Trilism is not a solitary vision but a shared evolution.

Remember: There is no me, there is no you—we are one. We are Trilists.

Trilism Mission Statement

Trilism is a living philosophy dedicated to the elevation of the human spirit through the integration of mind, body, and soul. Rooted in six core virtues—Health, Integrity, Resilience, Empathy, Social Harmony, and Authenticity—Trilism empowers individuals to cultivate personal wholeness while contributing to a just, compassionate, and peaceful world.

We exist to inspire conscious living, ethical decision-making, and human evolution through inner transformation and social responsibility. We do not seek control, but alignment; not power, but presence. We believe that by nurturing the individual, we nurture the collective.

Our mission is to guide, embody, and share a way of life where each person can thrive in truth, live in balance, and lead by example—building a better world from within.

We are Trilists!

So, What Next and How It Spreads—PEACEFULLY! The Immunity of Trilism—Why It Cannot Be Corrupted for Violence

Induction

In the modern era of ideological distortion and information warfare, many philosophies and religions have suffered manipulation by those seeking power, dominance, or legitimacy for violence. Trilism stands uniquely resistant to such misuse. What follows is a foundational reflection titled "Trilist Defence Against Corruption," a safeguard designed to demonstrate why Trilism cannot be weaponized, distorted, or hijacked. For scholars, seekers, and adherents, this section serves as both shield and compass.

Trilist Defence Against Corruption

1. Ethical Self-Reflection and Accountability

Principle:

Trilism enshrines ethical self-reflection as a sacred duty. Everyone must act in harmony with its six cardinal virtues: Empathy, Integrity, Health, Resilience, Social Harmony, and Authenticity.

Safeguard Against Corruption:

Violence or manipulation would instantly contradict Empathy and Integrity, disqualifying the perpetrator as a true practitioner

The philosophy does not permit blind obedience—only conscious ethical alignment.

Accountability is personal, continual, and internalized. No external force can dictate or justify actions that stray from these virtues.

2. Absence of Centralized Authority

Principle:

Trilism is decentralized. There is no pope, imam, prophet, or singular institution empowered to issue edicts or directives.

Safeguard Against Corruption

Without a leader to corrupt, there is no pyramid of power to seize.

Interpretive plurality ensures any radical misinterpretation will be checked by others within the community.

The community, united by shared values and virtues, becomes the ethical anchor—not any individual leader or hierarchical structure.

3. Community and Shared Values as the Core

Principle:

The Trilist community is bound not by external rules, but by internalized virtues. These values transcend geographic, cultural, and political boundaries, offering a universal blueprint for ethical living.

Safeguard Against Corruption

The strength of Trilism lies in its inclusivity and adaptability. No one person or group has ultimate control over its direction.

When in doubt, the community's collective wisdom serves as the final arbitrator of ethical conduct.

If any group attempts to corrupt the philosophy for personal gain or violent purposes, the collective will resist and call for reflection and reform, preventing exploitation or divisiveness.

4. Living Framework, Not Fixed Dogma

Principle:

Trilism is not a static creed. It evolves through reflection, conversation, and pragmatic adaptation.

Safeguard Against Corruption

Its openness immunizes it from being turned into rigid doctrine.

Questions are welcomed; orthodoxy is alien.

Dogmatism and fundamentalism, which often fuel radicalism, cannot find a foothold. Trilism thrives on growth, dialogue, and the healthy exchange of ideas. Any attempt to enforce a fixed ideology runs counter to its core values of Authenticity and Resilience, which invite personal evolution and wisdom through engagement, not imposition.

5. No Sacred Texts to Distort

Principle:

There is no "holy book" in Trilism—only guiding principles subject to ethical reasoning.

Safeguard Against Corruption:

There is nothing to quote out of context to justify harm.

No divine mandates to coerce others.

No prophecies or commandments to exploit. In the absence of a literal text to wield, Trilism operates in the realm of human experience, lived truth, and reason. This approach ensures that the philosophy cannot be weaponized through selective interpretation, as it is rooted in ongoing ethical inquiry, not rigid, dogmatic authority.

6. Built-In Resistance to Extremism

Principle:

Extremism cannot thrive in an ecosystem defined by compassion, mutual understanding, and truthfulness.

Safeguard Against Corruption

Core virtues repel radicalism as a toxin.

Nonviolence is not a strategic choice—it is a moral necessity.

To act violently in Trilism is to act against Trilism. The very essence of Trilism is founded upon Empathy, Social Harmony, and Integrity, all of which inherently reject the divisiveness and violence that extremist ideologies foster. By emphasizing cooperation over division, and compassion over coercion, Trilism fosters a culture where extremism is not tolerated, nor does it find fertile ground to take root.

7. Transparent Intent and Open Ethos

Principle:

Trilism declares its values publicly. There is no hidden agenda, no coded ambitions.

Safeguard Against Corruption:

Deception becomes impossible when Authenticity and Honesty are core requirements.

Secretive cells or power-seeking factions cannot grow undetected.

Those who distort its message expose themselves by violating its essence. The transparency of Trilism's goals ensures that any attempt to corrupt its message or exploit its virtues will be plainly visible to all who share in its community. The openness of its ethos means that every practitioner carries the duty of protecting its integrity by living openly and truthfully. This eliminates the opportunity for subversive or authoritarian factions to manipulate the philosophy for selfish or harmful purposes.

Conclusion: A Philosophy Immune to Corruption

With the safeguards outlined in this framework, Trilism stands as a philosophy that is not easily co-opted, corrupted, or weaponized. Its decentralized nature, ethical foundations, and commitment to openness ensure that it remains a living, breathing guide for those seeking personal and collective evolution.

The continuous process of self-reflection, community-based leadership, and a deep commitment to non-violence protect Trilism from becoming anything other than a force for good. The virtues of Empathy, Integrity, Resilience, Authenticity, Social Harmony, and Health are not just principles—they are practical tools for navigating the complexities of human life in a peaceful and ethical manner.

As we move forward, Trilism will not be shaped by the hands of power-hungry individuals or groups, but by the hearts and minds of those who live its values, creating a ripple effect of peace and transformation.

We are not just followers—we are the first branches of a growing tree, each of us contributing to the beauty of its roots and the wisdom of its leaves.

We are Trilists. We are the flow of peace, integrity, and shared humanity.

Scholar's Appendix: How to Spread Trilism Peacefully

For philosophers, ethicists, and educators, the propagation of Trilism must follow its internal logic—peace, dialogue, and self-awareness. The following approaches form the scholarly transmission strategy:

1. Ethical Education, Not Evangelism

Principle:
Trilism must be introduced as a thought-provoking philosophy rather than a dogmatic movement.
Approach:

Teach Trilism through philosophical inquiry, not missionary zeal. The aim is to spark critical thinking and self-reflection, not to convert or recruit.

Focus on virtue ethics, comparative moral frameworks, and lived examples to demonstrate the practical applicability of Trilism in real life. By showing how Trilism aligns with universal human aspirations for well-being and integrity, educators invite others to engage without force or coercion.

Avoid claiming exclusivity or superiority. Trilism should be offered as a respectful invitation to reflection, not as the definitive truth over all other philosophies. The goal is not to replace other traditions but to complement them, allowing individuals to integrate what resonates most with their own experiences and values.

2. Academic Integration

Principle:

The scholarly transmission of Trilism is rooted in engagement with established academic disciplines, ensuring intellectual rigor and broad acceptance.

Approach:

Publish in journals of ethics, comparative religion, and political theory, positioning Trilism as a serious and thoughtful contribution to global philosophical discourse.

Host dialogues with scholars from diverse traditions—such as Stoicism, Confucianism, Kantian ethics, Existentialism and all other philosophers—to explore common threads, differences, and the intersections of their ideas. This cross-pollination not only broadens the scope of Trilism but also enriches its understanding and applicability in modern contexts.

Encourage interdisciplinary studies that bridge the gap between philosophy, psychology, governance, and community-building. By weaving Trilism into the fabric of practical disciplines, it can be demonstrated as a usable framework for societal growth, personal development, and ethical decision-making.

3. Community Engagement

Principle:

Trilism thrives when its principles are lived out in community, where individuals can see its tangible benefits through action and interaction.

Approach:

Apply Trilism locally: in schools, cooperatives, and volunteer networks. Small-scale implementations allow for real-world applications and the cultivation of deeper relationships based on the philosophy's virtues.

Highlight civic ethics, empathy-based dialogue, and conflict resolution in action. Encourage practices that foster Social Harmony and

Resilience in community structures, proving that Trilism works not in theory but in everyday situations.

Let results, not slogans, become the testimony of its value. Invite others to observe and experience the positive impact of living by Trilism, rather than relying on empty promises or abstract claims.

Encourage active personal reflection and ongoing community-building as key elements in living Trilism. Practitioners should not simply accept its tenets but engage actively with the philosophy, reflecting on how it can improve their daily interactions, health, and sense of purpose. This active participation reinforces Trilism as a continuous, evolving journey, not a one-time acceptance.

4. Digital Transparency

Principle:

In the digital age, transparency, openness, and respect for privacy are essential to the responsible spread of any philosophy.

Approach:

Publish all tenets, critiques, and updates openly. To maintain the integrity of Trilism, it is essential that its development be visible and transparent to all. Regular updates and open access to philosophical discussions ensure a dynamic, evolving framework.

Maintain public forums for revision, challenge, and growth. Create platforms where individuals can express their interpretations, ask questions, and contribute their insights. A thriving digital space of respectful dialogue invites diverse perspectives, preventing Trilism from becoming a rigid or closed system.

Use the internet to foster dialogue, not propaganda. Trilism must be spread through reasoned discussions and mutual respect, not through manipulation or mindless repetition of slogans. Social media, blogs, podcasts, and other digital platforms should serve as spaces for critical engagement rather than tools for one-sided messaging.

Uphold digital ethics. Ensure that the tools and platforms used to spread Trilism respect privacy, consent, and promote respectful dialogue. Avoid the exploitation or manipulation of personal data, and resist using technology to control or manipulate practitioners. The philosophy must remain true to its principles in every aspect, including its digital presence.

5. Ethical Resistance to Co-otation

Principle:

Trilism must remain free from exploitation, distortion, or hijacking by those with ulterior motives.

Approach:

Be vigilant against the distortion of Trilism by any state, institution, or group with ulterior motives. There are always risks that any powerful idea, if not carefully safeguarded, can be exploited for political, social, or financial gain.

Reaffirm the philosophy's core values and guard against its manipulation for harmful purposes. Any attempt to co-opt Trilism for violent, authoritarian, or exploitative purposes must be immediately recognized and resisted by the community of Trilists.

Maintain open communication channels to ensure that deviations from Trilism's core principles are addressed quickly and transparently. As the philosophy spreads, it is crucial that its community remains committed to self-awareness and accountability, ensuring that Trilism remains a peaceful, ethical framework for living.

6. Encouraging Personal Reflection

While spreading Trilism in academic, community, and digital spaces is vital, the most profound change happens in the personal realm. Trilism is not a philosophy of external dogma, but of internal transformation. The spread of Trilism begins with each individual who internalizes its six core virtues—Health, Integrity, Resilience, Empathy, Social Harmony, and Authenticity

Trilism encourages personal reflection through journaling, meditative practices, and deliberate contemplation of the virtues in action. It emphasizes self-accountability, asking each follower to question: How can I embody these virtues more fully today?

This introspective approach is vital because it reflects the principle that Trilism grows organically, not through forceful measures or external pressures. Each person who practices Trilism authentically is a living testament to its value, naturally drawing others to explore its virtues.

7. Avoiding Overzealous Evangelism

One of the greatest threats to any idea, even the most peaceful and virtuous, is the temptation to turn it into an evangelistic crusade. Trilism must remain free from the risk of zealotry. Therefore, its spread should always remain non-coercive, focusing on invitation rather than persuasion.

Encourage others to explore Trilism at their own pace. Invite them to reflect on the Six Virtues, share the Manifesto, and allow them to connect with the philosophy through their lived experience. It is important to remember that Trilism is about personal choice and growth, not about converting others to a singular worldview. Be mindful of how you present Trilism: let it be a gentle call, a pathway to a better life, rather than an obligation. The peaceful propagation of Trilism depends on this delicate balance of offering without pressuring. **It's an invitation, not an obligation.**

8. Ethical Use of Technology

In our modern era, digital platforms play a significant role in the spread of ideas. Trilism must make use of these platforms without falling into the trap of exploitative digital marketing or misleading practices.

Transparency is key. All teachings, updates, and reflections should be accessible and open. Platforms like blogs, forums, podcasts, and social media can serve as useful tools to invite honest, reflective discussions. However, it's important to avoid any manipulative tactics—no clickbait, no manipulation of algorithms to force Trilism's ideas on others.

Create a digital space where all can engage respectfully with the philosophy, share their experiences, and debate ideas openly. This should be a space for constructive dialogue, not propaganda. We must uphold the same core principles of authenticity, empathy, and social harmony in the virtual world as we do in the real world.

Final Reflections: The Heart of Trilism

As we conclude this book, the essence of Trilism remains simple yet profound: a way of life grounded in the integration of mind, body, and soul, guided by six core virtues. These virtues are the heartbeat of the philosophy, and it is through their practice that Trilism takes root in the hearts and lives of individuals, transforming them from the inside out.

Trilism is not a rigid set of rules or a static dogma. It is a living, breathing philosophy that evolves with those who embrace it. It grows through dialogue, reflection, and mutual understanding. The true power of Trilism lies not in its spread through force or domination but in the quiet example of those who choose to live it authentically.

We must also acknowledge that the philosophy is not limited to those who call themselves "Trilists" but can, in fact, be a universal guide for anyone seeking a life of balance, integrity, and compassionate action. Trilism offers a model of ethical living that transcends traditional divisions, a philosophy rooted in the common good.

Conclusion: A Call to Action

The final invitation is not just to believe in Trilism but to live it—to embody the Six Virtues in daily life and become a living testament to the philosophy's transformative power. You are not just a follower but a participant in an ongoing, organic evolution of ethical living.

By adopting Trilism, you do not seek to separate yourself from others but to connect more deeply with them. You become an active part of a growing community—one that nurtures itself through collective virtue and shared responsibility.

Trilism is peace, it is action, it is love. It's not just a philosophy; it's a idea, and it begins within each of us.

A Vision for the Future: The Ripple Effect

As each Trilist adopts and practices the Six Virtues, their actions ripple outwards, influencing the world in ways both visible and subtle. Every kind act, every decision rooted in empathy, every effort to reconcile differences, every moment spent in self-reflection contributes to the collective growth of humanity.

Imagine a world where communities, businesses, governments, and individuals live in harmony with these virtues—where people actively work to improve not only their own lives but the lives of those around them. Imagine a society not defined by division or violence but by compassion, resilience, and authenticity.

That is the future Trilism envisions. It is not an ideal; it is a possibility—a reality that begins with you, the reader, the Trilist.

Appendix: The Six Virtues of Trilism

For ease of reference, we close with a summary of the Six Virtues of Trilism, along with practical tips on how to embody them in daily life.

1. Health: Prioritize your well-being—physical, emotional, and mental. Strive for balance, listen to your body, and nurture your mind.
Daily Action: Practice self-care rituals (exercise, balanced diet, mindfulness).

2. Integrity: Uphold honesty, moral consistency, and truthfulness.
Daily Action: Speak your truth, live authentically, and maintain your commitments.

3. Resilience: Cultivate mental and emotional strength. Overcome challenges with grace and perseverance.

Daily Action: Face adversity with courage, learn from setbacks, and grow stronger.

4. Empathy: Develop a deep understanding of others' feelings and needs. Act with kindness and compassion.

Daily Action: Listen actively, offer support, and walk in others' shoes.

5. Social Harmony: Foster unity and peaceful coexistence. Work toward resolving conflicts with respect and understanding.

Daily Action: Mediate disagreements, promote cooperation, and nurture inclusive communities.

6. Authenticity: Live in alignment with your true self. Do not compromise your values for external validation.

Daily Action: Reflect on your actions, remain true to your principles, and express your true self

Final Words: The Trilist Journey

The journey of Trilism is lifelong. It is not a destination but a continual process of growth, reflection, and self-improvement. As you embark on this path, remember that there is no "me," there is no "you," there is only "we." Together, we are Trilists, united by our commitment to personal growth and collective flourishing.

Now, it's time for you to take your first step—not as a follower, but as an active, living embodiment of Trilism. The world is waiting for you to lead by example, to spread the light of this philosophy not through force or control, but through the peaceful, powerful force of example. We are Trilists!

If you seek to grace the world with culture and refinement,

To weave your life in the elegance of thought and action,

I offer you my humble masterpiece,

A guide to being cultured and refined,

Without the stain of arrogance.

It is a path to sophistication,

Not through superiority, but through humility.

A journey that elevates the soul,

Without distancing it from others.

My book is called – *How to be cultured and refined without being a snob!*

Your friend always,
Gerry

Now you free yourself from your chains.

www.ingramcontent.com/pod-product-compliance
Lightning Source LLC
Chambersburg PA
CBHW031445040426
42444CB00007B/974